VERTICAL REFLEX THERAPY (VRT) COMPENDIUM

Dr. James K. Ferguson

COPYRIGHT © 2024 by Dr. James K. Ferguson

TABLE OF CONTENTS

INTRODUCTION

Welcome to the world of Vertical Reflex Therapy (VRT), where healing meets innovation and balance is within reach. In this comprehensive handbook, it starts with the depths of VRT, a revolutionary approach to reflexology that has the power to transform your understanding of health and well-being.

The Evolution of Reflexology: Reflexology, an ancient healing art dating back thousands of years, has long been revered for its ability to stimulate the body's natural healing processes through pressure applied to specific reflex points. Traditional reflexology primarily focuses on the feet and hands in a horizontal position, but VRT takes this practice to new heights—literally.

A Shift in Perspective: The concept of VRT is simple yet profound: by applying pressure to the reflex points of the weight-bearing feet and hands in a vertical position, the body's response is enhanced, leading to deeper relaxation, quicker results, and a more profound sense of balance. This shift in perspective not only enhances the effectiveness of reflexology but also opens up new possibilities for holistic healing.

Benefits Beyond Measure: The benefits of VRT are vast and varied, ranging from pain management to stress relief, and from enhanced circulation to improved overall well-being. By understanding the principles and techniques of

VRT, you can tap into a powerful tool for self-care and healing that can be integrated into your daily life or professional practice.

What You'll Discover in This Compendium: This compendium is your comprehensive guide to VRT, offering a detailed exploration of its history, principles, and techniques. Whether you're a seasoned reflexology practitioner looking to expand your skills or a newcomer curious about the potential of VRT, this book will provide you with the knowledge and tools you need to unlock the full potential of this transformative therapy.

Embark on a Journey of Healing: As you embark on this journey through the world of VRT, I invite you to open your mind to new possibilities, embrace the power of holistic healing, and discover the key to balance and well-being. Together, let's unlock the potential of Vertical Reflex Therapy and embark on a path to a healthier, more balanced life.

Welcome to the world of VRT—where healing begins from the ground up.

CHAPTER 1

20 important things you should know about (VRT)

1. Vertical Reflex Therapy (VRT) is a form of reflexology that involves applying pressure to the feet in a weight-bearing position, which is believed to enhance the effectiveness of the treatment.

2. VRT is based on the principle that the feet are more responsive to treatment when the body's weight is placed on them.

3. The technique was developed by Lynne Booth in the 1990s and has gained popularity as an alternative therapy for various conditions.

4. VRT is often used to improve circulation, reduce pain and tension, and promote relaxation.

5. The therapy is typically performed with the client standing or sitting, allowing the practitioner to work on the feet more effectively.

6. VRT can be used as a standalone treatment or in conjunction with other therapies, such as massage or acupuncture.

7. The therapy is believed to stimulate the nerve endings in the feet, which can have a beneficial effect on the corresponding organs and systems in the body.

8. Some studies suggest that VRT may be effective in reducing pain and improving mobility in conditions such as arthritis and back pain.

9. VRT is considered safe for most people, but it may not be suitable for those with certain medical conditions, such as foot injuries or infections.

10. The therapy is usually performed by a trained practitioner who will assess the client's condition and tailor the treatment accordingly.

11. VRT sessions typically last between 30 and 60 minutes, depending on the client's needs and the practitioner's recommendations.

12. Many people find VRT to be a relaxing and enjoyable experience, with some reporting immediate improvements in their symptoms.

13. Like other forms of reflexology, VRT is based on the belief that the body has the ability to heal itself, and the therapy aims to support this natural healing process.

14. Some practitioners may use tools or devices to enhance the effectiveness of VRT, such as small sticks or rollers to apply pressure to specific points on the feet.

15. VRT is not intended to replace conventional medical treatment, but it can be used as a complementary therapy to support overall health and well-being.

16. The therapy is suitable for people of all ages, from children to the elderly, and can be beneficial for a wide range of conditions.

17. Some people may experience mild discomfort during or after a VRT session, but this is usually temporary and should subside quickly.

18. It is important to consult with a qualified practitioner before undergoing VRT, especially if you have any underlying health conditions or concerns.

19. VRT is often used as a preventive measure to maintain health and well-being, as well as to alleviate specific symptoms or conditions.

20. Overall, VRT is a gentle and non-invasive therapy that can have a positive impact on both physical and emotional health.

CHAPTER 2

Overview of Vertical Reflex Therapy (VRT)

Vertical Reflex Therapy (VRT) is a revolutionary approach to reflexology that is performed on the weight-bearing feet and hands in a vertical position. This unique technique was developed by Lynne Booth in the early 1990s and has since gained popularity for its effectiveness in enhancing the benefits of traditional reflexology.

The concept of VRT is based on the theory that applying pressure to the reflex points of the feet and hands in a weight-bearing position can have a more profound effect on the body's systems. By stimulating these reflex points, VRT aims to improve circulation, release tension, and promote relaxation, leading to a wide range of health benefits.

One of the key principles of VRT is the idea that the body's response to reflexology can be enhanced when the reflex points are worked on in a vertical position. This is believed to be due to the increased gravitational pressure on the reflex points, which can stimulate a stronger response from the nervous system.

VRT is often used as a complementary therapy to traditional reflexology and is commonly used to help alleviate a variety of health issues, including back pain, digestive disorders, and stress-related conditions. It is also used as a preventive measure to promote overall health and well-being.

In summary, Vertical Reflex Therapy is a unique and effective approach to reflexology that offers a range of benefits for both the body and mind. By working on the reflex points of the feet and hands in a weight-bearing position, VRT can help improve circulation, release tension, and promote relaxation, leading to improved health and well-being.

Benefits of Vertical Reflex Therapy (VRT)

Vertical Reflex Therapy (VRT) offers a range of benefits for both physical and emotional well-being.

Some of the key benefits include:

1. Enhanced Reflexology Response: Working on the reflex points of the feet and hands in a weight-bearing position can enhance the body's response to reflexology, leading to quicker results and deeper relaxation.

2. Improved Circulation: By stimulating the reflex points, VRT can help improve circulation, which is essential for overall health and well-being.

3. Pain Relief: VRT is often used to help alleviate pain, particularly in the back, neck, and joints. It can also be effective for conditions such as arthritis and fibromyalgia.

4. Stress Reduction: The deep relaxation induced by VRT can help reduce stress and anxiety, promoting a sense of calm and well-being.

5. Enhanced Energy Levels: Many people find that VRT helps increase their energy levels and improves their overall sense of vitality.

6. Improved Sleep: VRT can help promote better sleep by inducing a state of deep relaxation.

7. Detoxification: Some practitioners believe that VRT can help stimulate the body's natural detoxification processes, aiding in the removal of toxins from the body.

8. Balancing Body Systems: By working on the reflex points, VRT aims to balance the body's systems, promoting overall health and well-being.

Principles of Vertical Reflex Therapy (VRT)

The principles of VRT are based on the same principles as traditional reflexology, with some key differences due to the weight-bearing aspect. **Some of the key principles of VRT include:**

1. Weight-Bearing Position: VRT is performed with the client standing or sitting, which is believed to enhance the body's response to the therapy.

2. Reflex Points: VRT focuses on stimulating the reflex points of the feet and hands, which are believed to correspond to different organs and systems of the body.

3. Enhanced Nervous System Response: The weight-bearing aspect of VRT is thought to stimulate a stronger response from the nervous system, leading to enhanced healing effects.

4. Integration with Traditional Reflexology: VRT is often used in conjunction with traditional reflexology techniques to enhance the overall effectiveness of the therapy.

5. Holistic Approach: Like traditional reflexology, VRT takes a holistic approach to health, treating the whole person rather than just the symptoms of a particular condition.

In summary, Vertical Reflex Therapy offers a range of benefits for both physical and emotional well-being. By stimulating the reflex points of the feet and hands in a weight-bearing position, VRT can help improve circulation, reduce pain and stress, and promote overall health and well-being.

Brief History and Development of Vertical Reflex Therapy (VRT)

Vertical Reflex Therapy (VRT) was developed by Lynne Booth, a reflexologist based in the United Kingdom, in the early 1990s. Booth had been practicing traditional reflexology for many years when she began to experiment with a new approach that involved working on the reflex points of the feet and hands in a weight-bearing position.

Booth's inspiration for VRT came from her observations that reflexology seemed to be more effective when the client was standing or sitting, rather than lying down. She hypothesized that the gravitational pressure on the reflex points in a weight-bearing position could stimulate a stronger response from the nervous system, leading to enhanced healing effects.

After refining her techniques through years of practice and research, Booth began teaching VRT to other reflexologists and health practitioners. The therapy quickly gained popularity for its effectiveness in treating a wide range of conditions, from back pain to digestive disorders.

Today, VRT is practiced by reflexologists around the world and is recognized as a valuable complement to traditional reflexology. Its unique approach and focus on the weight-bearing aspect set it apart from other forms of reflexology, making it a popular choice for those seeking a holistic approach to health and well-being.

In summary, Vertical Reflex Therapy is a relatively recent development in the field of reflexology, but its impact has been significant. Thanks to the pioneering work of Lynne Booth, VRT has helped countless people find relief from pain, stress, and other health issues, and continues to be a valuable tool for promoting overall health and well-being.

How Vertical Reflex Therapy (VRT) Complements Traditional Reflexology

Vertical Reflex Therapy (VRT) and traditional reflexology are both based on the principle that there are reflex points on the feet and hands that correspond to different organs and systems of the body. While they share this fundamental principle, VRT offers a unique approach that complements traditional reflexology in several ways:

1. Enhanced Reflex Response: One of the key ways that VRT complements traditional reflexology is by enhancing the body's response to the therapy. By working on the reflex points in a weight-bearing position, VRT is believed to stimulate a stronger response from the nervous system, leading to quicker results and deeper relaxation.

2. Quicker Results: Many practitioners and clients report that VRT can produce quicker results than traditional reflexology, particularly for acute conditions or pain relief. The weight-bearing aspect of VRT is thought to increase the effectiveness of the therapy, leading to faster healing.

3. Deeper Relaxation: The vertical position used in VRT can also lead to a deeper sense of relaxation for the client. This deep relaxation can help reduce stress and tension in the body, promoting a greater sense of well-being.

4. Comprehensive Approach: VRT offers a comprehensive approach to reflexology by incorporating techniques that address both the weight-bearing and non-weight-bearing reflex points. This comprehensive approach can lead to a more balanced and effective treatment.

5. Integration with Traditional Reflexology: VRT is often used in conjunction with traditional reflexology techniques to provide a more holistic treatment. Practitioners may use VRT to complement their traditional reflexology practice, offering clients a more diverse range of options for their health and well-being.

In summary, Vertical Reflex Therapy offers a unique and effective approach to reflexology that complements traditional techniques. By working on the reflex points in a weight-bearing position, VRT can enhance the body's response to reflexology, leading to quicker results, deeper relaxation, and a more comprehensive treatment.

CHAPTER 3

Understanding Reflexology Basics

Reflexology is a holistic therapy based on the principle that there are reflex points on the feet, hands, and ears that correspond to every part, gland, and organ of the body. By applying pressure to these reflex points, reflexologists believe they can stimulate the body's natural healing processes and promote balance and well-being.

History and Origins

Reflexology has ancient roots, with evidence of similar practices found in ancient Egypt, China, and India. Modern reflexology, however, is primarily based on the work of two American doctors, William H. Fitzgerald and Edwin Bowers, who developed the zone therapy theory in the early 20th century. This theory divides the body into ten zones, with each zone corresponding to specific areas on the feet, hands, and ears.

Principles of Reflexology

Reflexology is based on several key principles:

1. Reflex Points: Reflexologists believe that the reflex points on the feet, hands, and ears are connected to specific organs, glands, and body parts through energy pathways or zones. By applying pressure to these reflex points, they can stimulate the flow of energy and promote healing in the corresponding areas of the body.

2. Energy Flow: Reflexology is based on the concept of energy flow or life force, known as Qi (pronounced "chee") in traditional Chinese medicine. By unblocking and balancing the flow of energy through the body, reflexologists aim to promote health and well-being.

3. Homeostasis: Reflexology is believed to help the body achieve a state of homeostasis, or balance, by stimulating the body's natural healing mechanisms. This can help improve circulation, reduce stress, and promote relaxation.

Benefits of Reflexology

Reflexology is often used to:

- Reduce stress and tension

- Improve circulation
- Alleviate pain and discomfort
- Boost the immune system
- Improve sleep
- Enhance overall well-being

Reflexology is a gentle and non-invasive therapy that can be used to promote health and well-being. Whether used on its own or as a complement to other treatments, reflexology offers a holistic approach to healing that focuses on the body's natural ability to heal itself.

The Concept of Reflexology

Reflexology is a holistic healing practice based on the belief that specific areas on the feet, hands, and ears correspond to different organs and systems of the body. By applying pressure to these areas, reflexologists believe they can stimulate the body's natural healing process and promote overall well-being.

Key Principles of Reflexology:

1. Reflex Points: Reflexologists divide the body into zones and believe that there are reflex points within these zones that correspond to specific organs, glands, and body parts. By applying pressure to these reflex points, they aim to stimulate energy flow and promote healing in the corresponding areas of the body.

2. Energy Flow: Reflexology is based on the concept of energy flow within the body. It is believed that imbalances in this energy flow can lead to illness and that by stimulating the reflex points, balance can be restored, promoting health and well-being.

3. Holistic Approach: Reflexology takes a holistic approach to healing, treating the whole person rather than just the symptoms of a particular condition. It aims to address imbalances in the body and promote overall health and well-being.

How Reflexology Works

Reflexologists use their hands to apply pressure to the reflex points on the feet, hands, or ears. This pressure is thought to stimulate nerve endings, which then send signals to the brain to relax corresponding areas of the body. Reflexology is believed to help improve circulation, reduce stress, and promote relaxation, which can in turn help the body heal itself.

How Reflexology Affects the Body

Reflexology is believed to affect the body in several ways, primarily through the stimulation of reflex points on the feet, hands, and ears. **Here's a closer look at how reflexology is thought to impact the body:**

1. Stimulation of Nerve Endings: Reflexology involves applying pressure to specific reflex points, which are believed to stimulate nerve endings. These nerve endings then send signals to the brain, which can have various effects on the body.

2. Relaxation Response: One of the most well-documented effects of reflexology is its ability to induce a state of deep relaxation. This can help reduce stress and tension in the body, leading to a sense of calm and well-being.

3. Improved Circulation: By stimulating the reflex points, reflexology is thought to improve blood flow to the corresponding areas of the body. This can help improve circulation, which is essential for overall health and well-being.

4. Pain Relief: Reflexology is often used to help alleviate pain, particularly in the feet, hands, and head. By stimulating the reflex points, reflexologists believe they can help reduce pain and discomfort in the corresponding areas of the body.

5. Balancing Body Systems: Reflexology is based on the principle that the body is made up of interconnected systems that must be in balance for optimal health. By working on the reflex points, reflexologists aim to balance the body's systems, promoting overall health and well-being.

6. Detoxification: Some practitioners believe that reflexology can help stimulate the body's natural detoxification processes, aiding in the removal of toxins from the body.

7. Boosting the Immune System: Reflexology is thought to help boost the immune system by reducing stress and promoting relaxation, which can in turn help the body fight off illness and disease.

In summary, reflexology is believed to affect the body in a variety of ways, primarily through the stimulation of reflex points on the feet, hands, and ears. While more research is needed to fully understand how reflexology works, many people find it to be a relaxing and effective way to support their overall health and well-being.

Differences Between Traditional Reflexology and Vertical Reflex Therapy (VRT)

1. Body Position:

- Traditional Reflexology: Practiced with the client lying down or seated in a relaxed position.
- VRT: Practiced with the client in a weight-bearing position, either standing or

sitting, to enhance the body's response to the therapy.

2. Reflex Points:

- Traditional Reflexology: Focuses on all reflex points on the feet, hands, and ears.
- VRT: Focuses primarily on the weight-bearing reflex points on the feet and hands, which are believed to be more responsive and effective.

3. Pressure and Technique:

- Traditional Reflexology: Uses thumb, finger, and hand techniques to apply pressure to reflex points.
- VRT: Uses a combination of thumb, finger, and hand techniques, often with more emphasis on the weight-bearing

reflex points and a firmer pressure due to the standing or seated position.

4. Speed and Intensity:

- Traditional Reflexology: Techniques are often performed at a slower pace with varying degrees of pressure.
- VRT: Techniques are often performed at a quicker pace and with more intensity, aiming to achieve quicker results.

5. Depth of Relaxation:

- Traditional Reflexology: Can induce a deep state of relaxation.
- VRT: Often reported to induce a deeper state of relaxation due to the increased pressure and stimulation of the weight-bearing reflex points.

6. Application and Integration:

- Traditional Reflexology: Can be used as a standalone therapy or integrated with other complementary therapies.
- VRT: Can be used as a standalone therapy or integrated with traditional reflexology to enhance its effectiveness.

7. Focus and Scope:

- Traditional Reflexology: Focuses on the entire body and its systems, aiming to promote overall health and well-being.
- VRT: Focuses more on specific areas of the body through the weight-bearing reflex points, with a focus on enhancing

circulation, reducing pain, and promoting relaxation.

In summary, while both traditional reflexology and VRT share the same fundamental principles, they differ in their approach, techniques, and focus. VRT is a specialized form of reflexology that offers unique benefits and is particularly effective for those looking for a more intensive and targeted treatment.

How Vertical Reflex Therapy (VRT) Can Enhance the Benefits of Reflexology

Vertical Reflex Therapy (VRT) is a specialized form of reflexology that is believed to enhance the benefits of traditional reflexology in several ways:

1. Increased Pressure and Stimulation: The weight-bearing aspect of VRT allows for greater pressure to be applied to the reflex points, which can lead to increased stimulation of the nervous system. This increased pressure and stimulation are believed to enhance the body's response to the therapy, leading to quicker results and deeper relaxation.

2. Improved Circulation: The vertical position used in VRT is thought to improve circulation by allowing for better blood flow to the feet and hands. This improved circulation can help promote healing and reduce pain and discomfort in the corresponding areas of the body.

3. Deeper Relaxation: Many people find that VRT induces a deeper state of relaxation compared to traditional reflexology. This deep relaxation can help reduce stress and tension in the body, promoting a greater sense of well-being.

4. Targeted Treatment: VRT focuses primarily on the weight-bearing reflex points on the feet and hands, which are believed to be more responsive and effective. This targeted approach allows for a more intensive and focused treatment, making it particularly effective for addressing specific health issues.

5. Quicker Results: Due to its increased pressure and stimulation, VRT is often reported to produce quicker results than traditional reflexology. Many people find relief from pain and discomfort after just a few sessions of VRT.

6. Integration with Traditional Reflexology:
VRT can be used in conjunction with traditional reflexology techniques to enhance the overall effectiveness of the therapy. By combining these two approaches, practitioners can offer a more comprehensive and personalized treatment to their clients.

In summary, Vertical Reflex Therapy offers a unique and effective way to enhance the benefits of traditional reflexology. By applying pressure to the reflex points in a weight-bearing position, VRT can stimulate the body's natural healing processes, improve circulation, reduce stress, and promote overall well-being.

CHAPTER 4

The Fundamentals of Vertical Reflex Therapy (VRT)

Vertical Reflex Therapy (VRT) is a specialized form of reflexology that is practiced with the client in a weight-bearing position, either standing or sitting. This unique approach is believed to enhance the effectiveness of traditional reflexology by increasing the pressure and stimulation on the reflex points of the feet and hands.

Here are the key fundamentals of VRT:

1. Weight-Bearing Position: Unlike traditional reflexology, which is typically performed with the client lying down, VRT is performed with the client in a weight-bearing position. This allows for greater pressure to be applied to the reflex points, which is believed to enhance the body's response to the therapy.

2. Focus on Reflex Points: VRT focuses primarily on the weight-bearing reflex points on the feet and hands. These reflex points are believed to be more responsive and effective when stimulated in a weight-bearing position.

3. Quick Techniques: VRT techniques are often performed at a quicker pace than traditional reflexology, with shorter, more intense movements. This is thought to achieve quicker results and deeper relaxation.

4. Integration with Traditional Reflexology: While VRT is a distinct form of reflexology, it can be integrated with traditional techniques to enhance the overall effectiveness of the therapy. Practitioners may use VRT to complement their traditional reflexology practice, offering clients a more diverse range of options for their health and well-being.

5. Benefits: VRT is believed to offer a range of benefits, including improved circulation, reduced stress and tension, and enhanced relaxation. Many people find VRT to be particularly effective for addressing specific health issues and promoting overall well-being.

6. Professional Training: Due to its specialized nature, VRT requires specific training for practitioners. Many reflexology schools and organizations offer courses in VRT for those looking to expand their skills and knowledge in this area.

In summary, Vertical Reflex Therapy is a unique and effective approach to reflexology that offers several key advantages over traditional techniques. By focusing on the weight-bearing reflex points and applying pressure in a specific manner, VRT can enhance the benefits of reflexology and provide a more targeted and intensive treatment for clients.

The Theory Behind Vertical Reflex Therapy (VRT)

Vertical Reflex Therapy (VRT) is based on several key principles that differentiate it from traditional reflexology. These principles are rooted in the belief that reflex points on the feet and hands correspond to different organs and systems of the body, and that applying pressure to these reflex points can stimulate the body's natural healing processes.

Here is an overview of the theory behind VRT:

1. Weight-Bearing Reflex Points: VRT focuses primarily on the weight-bearing reflex points on the feet and hands. These reflex points are believed to be more responsive and effective when stimulated in a weight-bearing position, such as when the client is standing or sitting.

2. Enhanced Reflex Response: The weight-bearing aspect of VRT is thought to enhance the body's response to the therapy. By applying pressure to the reflex points in a weight-bearing position, VRT is believed to stimulate a stronger response from the nervous system, leading to quicker results and deeper relaxation.

3. Zone Theory: VRT is based on the zone therapy theory, which divides the body into ten vertical zones, with each zone corresponding to specific areas on the feet, hands, and ears. By applying pressure to these zones, reflexologists believe they can stimulate energy flow and promote healing in the corresponding areas of the body.

4. Energy Flow: Like traditional reflexology, VRT is based on the concept of energy flow within the body. It is believed that imbalances in this energy flow can lead to illness, and that by stimulating the reflex points, balance can be restored, promoting health and well-being.

5. Integration with Traditional Reflexology: While VRT is a distinct form of reflexology, it can be integrated with traditional techniques to enhance the overall effectiveness of the therapy. Practitioners may use VRT to complement their traditional reflexology practice, offering clients a more comprehensive and personalized treatment.

In summary, Vertical Reflex Therapy is based on the theory that applying pressure to specific reflex points on the feet and hands can stimulate the body's natural healing processes and promote overall health and well-being. By focusing on the weight-bearing reflex points and applying pressure in a specific manner, VRT offers a unique and effective approach to reflexology that can provide a range of benefits for clients.

How Vertical Reflex Therapy (VRT) Works on the Weight-Bearing Feet and Hands

Vertical Reflex Therapy (VRT) is a unique form of reflexology that is practiced with the client in a weight-bearing position, either standing or sitting. This approach is believed to enhance the effectiveness of the therapy by increasing the pressure and stimulation on the reflex points of the feet and hands.

Here is how VRT works on the weight-bearing feet and hands:

1. Increased Pressure: The weight-bearing aspect of VRT allows for greater pressure to be applied to the reflex points on the feet and hands. This increased pressure is believed to stimulate the nerve endings more effectively, leading to a stronger response from the nervous system.

2. Enhanced Stimulation: By applying pressure to the reflex points in a weight-bearing position, VRT is thought to enhance the stimulation of the reflex points. This increased stimulation is believed to promote the flow of energy and blood circulation to the corresponding areas of the body.

3. Quicker Results: Many practitioners and clients report that VRT can produce quicker results than traditional reflexology. The increased pressure and stimulation on the weight-bearing reflex points are believed to lead to quicker healing and deeper relaxation.

4. Deeper Relaxation: The pressure and stimulation applied during VRT can induce a deeper state of relaxation compared to traditional reflexology. This deep relaxation can help reduce stress and tension in the body, promoting a greater sense of well-being.

5. Balancing Body Systems: VRT aims to balance the body's systems by working on the reflex points in a weight-bearing position. This balanced approach is believed to promote overall health and well-being by stimulating the body's natural healing processes.

6. Integration with Traditional Reflexology: VRT can be integrated with traditional reflexology techniques to provide a more comprehensive treatment. Practitioners may use VRT to complement their traditional reflexology practice, offering clients a more diverse range of options for their health and well-being.

In summary, Vertical Reflex Therapy works on the weight-bearing feet and hands by applying pressure and stimulation to the reflex points in a specific manner. This unique approach is believed to enhance the effectiveness of the therapy and provide a range of benefits for clients, including quicker results, deeper relaxation, and overall health and well-being.

Benefits of Vertical Reflexology (VRT) versus Horizontal Reflexology

Vertical Reflex Therapy (VRT) and horizontal reflexology (traditional reflexology) both offer unique benefits, and the choice between them may depend on individual preferences and health needs.

Here are some key benefits of each:

1. Enhanced Stimulation: VRT is believed to provide more intense stimulation to the reflex points due to the weight-bearing position, potentially leading to quicker results and deeper relaxation.

2. Deeper Relaxation: Many people find that VRT induces a deeper state of relaxation compared to traditional reflexology, which can help reduce stress and tension more effectively.

3. Improved Circulation: The weight-bearing aspect of VRT is thought to improve circulation in the feet and hands, which can promote healing and reduce pain and discomfort.

4. Targeted Treatment: VRT focuses primarily on the weight-bearing reflex points, allowing for a more targeted and intensive treatment that may be particularly effective for specific health issues.

Horizontal Reflexology (Traditional Reflexology):

1. Comfort: Some people may find traditional reflexology more comfortable than VRT, as it is typically practiced with the client lying down or seated in a relaxed position.

2. Relaxation: Traditional reflexology can also induce a deep state of relaxation, which can help reduce stress and promote overall well-being.

3. Integration with Other Therapies: Traditional reflexology is well-established and can be easily integrated with other complementary therapies, offering a more holistic approach to health and well-being.

4. Flexibility: Traditional reflexology can be adapted to suit individual preferences and needs, making it a versatile therapy that can be customized for each client.

In summary, both VRT and traditional reflexology offer unique benefits and can be effective in promoting health and well-being. The choice between them may depend on individual preferences, health needs, and goals for treatment.

CHAPTER 5

Techniques and Application of Vertical Reflex Therapy (VRT)

Vertical Reflex Therapy (VRT) is a specialized form of reflexology that is practiced with the client in a weight-bearing position, either standing or sitting. This unique approach allows for greater pressure to be applied to the reflex points on the feet and hands, leading to enhanced stimulation and potentially quicker results.

Here are the key techniques and application of VRT:

1. Thumb Walking: Practitioners use their thumbs to walk across the reflex points on the feet and hands, applying firm pressure to stimulate the nerve endings. This technique is believed to promote energy flow and improve circulation to the corresponding areas of the body.

2. Finger Walking: In addition to thumb walking, practitioners may also use their fingers to walk across the reflex points. This technique allows for more precise pressure to be applied to specific areas, targeting areas of tension or discomfort.

3. Rotation: Practitioners may use a rotating motion with their thumbs or fingers to further stimulate the reflex points. This technique is believed to help release tension and promote relaxation in the corresponding areas of the body.

4. Reflexology Tools: Some practitioners use reflexology tools, such as wooden or metal probes, to apply pressure to the reflex points. These tools can help provide a more targeted and intensive treatment, particularly for areas that are difficult to reach with the hands.

5. Integration with Traditional Reflexology: VRT can be integrated with traditional reflexology techniques to provide a more comprehensive treatment. Practitioners may combine VRT with horizontal reflexology techniques, such as thumb walking and finger walking, to enhance the overall effectiveness of the therapy.

6. Application: VRT is typically practiced in short sessions, with the client standing or sitting in a relaxed position. Practitioners apply pressure to the reflex points on the feet and hands using their thumbs, fingers, or reflexology tools, focusing on the weight-bearing reflex points for maximum effect.

In summary, Vertical Reflex Therapy uses a combination of thumb walking, finger walking, rotation, and reflexology tools to stimulate the reflex points on the feet and hands. This unique approach allows for greater pressure to be applied to the reflex points, leading to enhanced stimulation and potentially quicker results.

Preparation and Setup for a Vertical Reflex Therapy (VRT) Session

Preparing for a Vertical Reflex Therapy (VRT) session involves creating a comfortable and conducive environment for the client to receive the therapy.

Here are the key steps involved in preparing for a VRT session:

1. Consultation: Begin the session with a consultation to discuss the client's health history, any specific concerns or areas of discomfort, and their goals for the session. This information will help tailor the treatment to meet the client's individual needs.

2. Setting: Choose a quiet and comfortable space for the session, free from distractions. Ensure that the room is warm and well-ventilated, with soft lighting and relaxing music if desired.

3. Seating Arrangement: For a seated VRT session, provide a comfortable chair for the client to sit in. The chair should provide adequate support and allow the client to sit in a relaxed position with their feet flat on the floor.

4. Footrest: If the client is standing for the session, provide a sturdy footrest for them to stand on. The footrest should be at a comfortable height and angle to allow the client to maintain their balance while receiving the therapy.

5. Equipment: Gather any equipment you will need for the session, such as reflexology tools, towels, and cushions. Have these items readily available for easy access during the session.

6. Preparation of the Feet: Before beginning the session, ensure that the client's feet are clean and dry. You may also offer them the option to soak their feet in warm water with Epsom salts or essential oils to relax and soften the skin.

7. Explanation of the Process: Take a few moments to explain the VRT process to the client, including what to expect during the session and any sensations they may experience. This will help them feel more comfortable and relaxed during the treatment.

8. Comfort and Support: Throughout the session, ensure that the client is comfortable and supported. Offer cushions or blankets as needed to help them relax and maintain a comfortable position.

By following these steps, you can create a comfortable and supportive environment for a VRT session, allowing the client to fully benefit from the therapy.

Step-by-Step Guide to Performing Vertical Reflex Therapy (VRT)

Performing Vertical Reflex Therapy (VRT) involves applying pressure to the reflex points on the weight-bearing feet and hands while the client is in a standing or seated position.

Here is a step-by-step guide to performing VRT:

1. Preparation:

- Set up a comfortable and quiet environment for the session.
- Ensure that the client's feet and hands are clean and dry.
- Have all necessary equipment, such as reflexology tools and towels, ready for use.

2. Consultation:

- Begin the session with a brief consultation to discuss the client's health history and any specific concerns or areas of discomfort.

- Explain the VRT process to the client and answer any questions they may have.

3. Seating Arrangement:

- For a seated session, provide a comfortable chair for the client to sit in with their feet flat on the floor.
- For a standing session, provide a sturdy footrest for the client to stand on.

4. Positioning:

- Position yourself in front of the client, facing their feet or hands.
- Ensure that you are in a comfortable position to apply pressure to the reflex points.

5. Thumb Walking:

- Begin by using your thumbs to walk across the reflex points on the client's feet or hands.

- Apply firm but gentle pressure to each reflex point, focusing on areas of tension or discomfort.

- Use a vertical motion, moving from the base to the top of the foot or hand.

6. Finger Walking:

- After thumb walking, you can use your fingers to walk across the reflex points, applying pressure in a similar manner.

- Use your fingers to target specific areas or reflex points that may require more attention.

7. Rotation:

- Use a rotating motion with your thumbs or fingers to further stimulate the reflex points.
- This can help release tension and promote relaxation in the corresponding areas of the body.

8. Reflexology Tools:

- If you are using reflexology tools, such as wooden or metal probes, apply them to the reflex points with gentle pressure.
- These tools can help provide a more targeted and intensive treatment.

9. Completion:

- Continue the VRT session for the desired length of time, typically 20-30 minutes per session.

- End the session with a gentle massage of the feet or hands to help the client relax.

10. Post-Session:

- After the session, offer the client water and encourage them to rest and relax.
- Provide any additional advice or recommendations for self-care between sessions.

By following this step-by-step guide, you can perform Vertical Reflex Therapy (VRT) effectively and provide your clients with a relaxing and beneficial experience.

Special Considerations and Modifications for Different Conditions in Vertical Reflex Therapy (VRT)

1. Pregnancy:

- Avoid using strong pressure on reflex points associated with the reproductive organs.
- Focus on points that can help alleviate common pregnancy discomforts, such as nausea, back pain, and swollen ankles.

2. Circulatory Issues:

- Use gentle pressure and avoid vigorous massage techniques.

- Focus on points that can help improve circulation, such as those associated with the heart and circulatory system.

3. Diabetes:

- Avoid using strong pressure, as people with diabetes may have reduced sensation in their feet.
- Focus on points that can help improve circulation and nerve function, such as those associated with the feet and legs.

4. Arthritis:

- Use gentle pressure and avoid placing too much weight on the joints.
- Focus on points that can help reduce inflammation and improve joint mobility.

5. Neuropathy:

- Use very light pressure, as people with neuropathy may have reduced sensation in their feet and hands.
- Focus on points that can help improve nerve function and circulation, such as those associated with the feet and hands.

6. Injuries:

- Avoid applying pressure to areas that are injured or inflamed.
- Focus on points that can help promote healing and reduce pain, such as those associated with the injured area.

7. Chronic Conditions:

- Modify the pressure and intensity of the treatment based on the individual's comfort level.

- Focus on points that can help alleviate symptoms and improve overall health and well-being.

8. Medication and Medical History:

- Always ask about the client's medication and medical history before starting the treatment.
- Modify the treatment based on any contraindications or special considerations related to their health condition.

9. Client Feedback:

- Throughout the session, communicate with the client and ask for feedback on the pressure and technique.
- Modify the treatment based on their feedback to ensure their comfort and safety.

10. Post-Session Care:

- Provide the client with any recommended self-care practices or exercises to complement the VRT treatment.
- Follow up with the client to assess their progress and make any necessary modifications to their treatment plan.

By considering these special considerations and modifications, you can adapt your Vertical Reflex Therapy (VRT) treatment to meet the unique needs of clients with different conditions, ensuring a safe and effective treatment experience.

CHAPTER 6

Integrating Vertical Reflex Therapy (VRT) into Your Practice

Integrating Vertical Reflex Therapy (VRT) into your practice can offer clients a unique and effective approach to reflexology.

Here are some steps to consider when integrating VRT into your practice:

1. Training and Certification:

- Obtain training and certification in VRT from a reputable organization.
- Ensure that you are knowledgeable and skilled in the techniques and principles of VRT before offering it to clients.

2. Client Education:

- Educate your clients about the benefits of VRT and how it differs from traditional reflexology.

- Explain the process and what they can expect during a VRT session.

3. Assessment and Treatment Planning:

- Conduct a thorough assessment of your client's health history and any specific concerns they may have.

- Develop a treatment plan that includes VRT techniques tailored to their individual needs.

4. Incorporating VRT into Sessions:

- Integrate VRT techniques into your reflexology sessions, focusing on the weight-bearing reflex points.

- Use a combination of thumb walking, finger walking, and rotation techniques to stimulate the reflex points.

5. Client Feedback and Communication:

- Encourage open communication with your clients during the session.
- Ask for feedback on the pressure and technique to ensure their comfort and satisfaction.

6. Follow-Up and Monitoring:

- Follow up with your clients after the session to assess their progress and address any concerns.
- Monitor their response to the treatment and make any necessary adjustments to their treatment plan.

7. Continuing Education and Development:

- Stay updated on the latest research and developments in VRT.

- Attend workshops and seminars to further develop your skills and knowledge in VRT.

8. Marketing and Promotion:

- Promote your VRT services to your existing clients and through marketing channels such as social media and your website.

- Highlight the benefits of VRT and how it can enhance their overall well-being.

By following these steps, you can effectively integrate Vertical Reflex Therapy (VRT) into your practice and offer clients a unique and beneficial form of reflexology.

How to Incorporate Vertical Reflex Therapy (VRT) into an Existing Reflexology Practice

Incorporating Vertical Reflex Therapy (VRT) into an existing reflexology practice can enhance the range of services you offer and provide clients with a unique and effective treatment option.

Here's how you can incorporate VRT into your practice:

1. Training and Certification:

- Obtain training and certification in VRT from a reputable organization.
- Ensure that you are knowledgeable and skilled in the techniques and principles of VRT before offering it to clients.

2. Assessment and Consultation:

- Conduct a thorough assessment of your clients' health history and reflexology needs.
- Discuss with them the benefits of VRT and how it can complement traditional reflexology.

3. Integrating VRT Techniques:

- Integrate VRT techniques into your reflexology sessions, focusing on the weight-bearing reflex points.
- Use thumb walking, finger walking, and rotation techniques to stimulate the reflex points.

4. Educating Clients:

- Educate your clients about VRT and how it differs from traditional reflexology.

- Explain the benefits of VRT and how it can enhance their overall well-being.

5. Client Feedback and Communication:

- Encourage open communication with your clients during the session.
- Ask for feedback on the pressure and technique to ensure their comfort and satisfaction.

6. Customizing Treatment Plans:

- Develop customized treatment plans for your clients that incorporate VRT techniques based on their individual needs.
- Modify the treatment plan as needed based on their feedback and progress.

7. Marketing and Promotion:

- Promote your VRT services to your existing clients and through marketing channels such as social media and your website.
- Highlight the benefits of VRT and how it can complement traditional reflexology.

8. Continuing Education and Development:

- Stay updated on the latest research and developments in VRT.
- Attend workshops and seminars to further develop your skills and knowledge in VRT.

By incorporating Vertical Reflex Therapy (VRT) into your existing reflexology practice, you can offer clients a unique and effective treatment option that can enhance their overall well-being.

Marketing and Promoting Vertical Reflex Therapy (VRT) Services

Marketing and promoting your VRT services can help you reach a wider audience and attract new clients to your practice.

Here are some strategies to consider:

1. Website and Online Presence:

- Create a dedicated page on your website for your VRT services, highlighting the benefits and explaining the process.
- Optimize your website for search engines (SEO) to improve visibility online.

- Consider creating a blog or articles related to VRT to provide valuable information to potential clients.

2. Social Media Marketing:

- Use social media platforms such as Facebook, Instagram, and Twitter to promote your VRT services.
- Share posts about the benefits of VRT, client testimonials, and special offers or promotions.
- Engage with your audience by responding to comments and messages promptly.

3. Networking and Partnerships:

- Network with other healthcare professionals, such as chiropractors, naturopaths, and massage therapists, who may refer clients to you for VRT.

- Consider partnering with wellness centers, spas, or gyms to offer VRT services to their clients.

4. Printed Materials:

- Create brochures or flyers that promote your VRT services and distribute them in local businesses or healthcare facilities.
- Consider placing ads in local newspapers or magazines that cater to health and wellness.

5. Workshops and Events:

- Host workshops or informational sessions about VRT to educate the community and attract potential clients.
- Participate in health fairs or community events to showcase your VRT services and connect with potential clients.

6. Client Referral Program:

- Implement a client referral program where existing clients can earn rewards or discounts for referring new clients to your VRT services.

- Encourage satisfied clients to leave reviews and testimonials that can be used in your marketing materials.

7. Professional Associations:

- Join professional associations related to reflexology and alternative medicine to connect with other practitioners and stay updated on industry trends.

- Consider becoming a certified VRT instructor to expand your reach and credibility in the field.

8. Collaborate with Influencers:

- Partner with influencers or bloggers in the health and wellness niche to promote your VRT services to their audience.

- Offer them a complimentary session in exchange for a review or social media post about their experience.

By implementing these marketing strategies, you can effectively promote your VRT services and attract new clients to your practice.

Case Studies and Success Stories of Vertical Reflex Therapy (VRT)

1. Case Study: Chronic Back Pain Relief:

- Client Profile: A 45-year-old office worker with chronic lower back pain.

- Treatment: Six sessions of VRT focusing on the weight-bearing reflex points of the feet.

- Results: After the sessions, the client reported a significant reduction in back pain and improved mobility. They were able to resume activities they had previously avoided due to pain.

2. Case Study: Insomnia and Stress Reduction:

- Client Profile: A 35-year-old teacher experiencing insomnia and high stress levels.

- Treatment: Eight sessions of VRT combined with relaxation techniques.

- Results: The client experienced improved sleep quality and reduced stress levels after the sessions. They reported feeling more relaxed and able to cope better with daily challenges.

3. Case Study: Digestive Issues Improvement:

- Client Profile: A 50-year-old woman with long-standing digestive issues.

- Treatment: Ten sessions of VRT focusing on reflex points related to the digestive system.

- Results: The client reported significant improvement in digestive symptoms, including reduced bloating and discomfort. They also experienced better appetite and digestion.

4. Success Story: Enhanced Well-being and Energy:

- Client Profile: A 55-year-old man looking to improve his overall well-being and energy levels.

- Treatment: Regular VRT sessions combined with lifestyle changes, including diet and exercise.

- Results: The client reported feeling more energetic and focused after starting VRT. He also noticed improvements in his mood and overall sense of well-being.

5. Success Story: Pain Management and Mobility:

- Client Profile: A 60-year-old woman with arthritis seeking pain relief and improved mobility.

- Treatment: VRT sessions focused on reflex points associated with pain management and joint health.

- Results: The client experienced reduced pain and stiffness in her joints, allowing her to move more freely and engage in daily activities with greater ease.

These case studies and success stories demonstrate the potential benefits of Vertical Reflex Therapy (VRT) for a variety of health conditions. Each client's experience is unique, and results may vary. However, these examples highlight the positive impact that VRT can have on physical and emotional well-being.

CHAPTER 7

Advanced VRT Concepts and Innovations

1. Zone Therapy Integration:

- Incorporating principles of zone therapy into VRT to target specific zones of the body through the feet and hands.

2. Meridian Reflexology:

- Applying VRT techniques to stimulate meridian lines in the body, based on traditional Chinese medicine principles.

3. Energy Work:

- Utilizing VRT to work with the body's energy systems, such as chakras, to promote balance and harmony.

4. Advanced Reflex Points:

- Exploring lesser-known reflex points on the feet and hands that correspond to specific organs or systems in the body.

5. VRT Protocols for Specific Conditions:

- Developing specialized VRT protocols for conditions such as chronic pain, autoimmune disorders, and neurological conditions.

6. VRT and Mental Health:

- Using VRT to support mental health by addressing stress, anxiety, and emotional imbalances through reflex points.

7. Research and Evidence-Based Practice:

- Conducting and participating in research studies to further validate the effectiveness of VRT and enhance its integration into mainstream healthcare.

8. VRT Technology:

- Exploring the use of technology, such as biofeedback devices or virtual reality, to enhance the effects of VRT and improve client outcomes.

9. VRT Training and Education:

- Developing advanced training programs and continuing education courses for reflexologists interested in expanding their knowledge and skills in VRT.

10. Integration with Other Modalities:

- Integrating VRT with other complementary modalities, such as aromatherapy, sound therapy, or massage, to create comprehensive treatment plans for clients.

These advanced concepts and innovations in Vertical Reflex Therapy (VRT) are pushing the boundaries of traditional reflexology and opening up new possibilities for its application in promoting health and well-being.

New Developments in Vertical Reflex Therapy (VRT) Research

1. Pain Management: Recent studies have shown that VRT can be effective in managing chronic pain conditions, such as lower back pain and arthritis, by stimulating reflex points associated with pain relief.

2. Stress Reduction: Research has demonstrated that VRT can help reduce stress levels and promote relaxation by stimulating reflex points that correspond to the nervous system and stress response.

3. Improved Circulation: Studies have indicated that VRT may improve circulation in the feet and hands, leading to better overall blood flow and oxygenation of tissues.

4. Enhanced Immune Function: Preliminary research suggests that VRT may have immune-boosting effects by stimulating reflex points associated with the lymphatic system and immune response.

5. Mental Health Benefits: Emerging research indicates that VRT may have positive effects on mental health, including reducing symptoms of anxiety and depression, by stimulating reflex points linked to emotional well-being.

6. Neurological Effects: Some studies suggest that VRT may have beneficial effects on neurological conditions, such as Parkinson's disease and multiple sclerosis, by stimulating reflex points that correspond to the central nervous system.

7. Integration with Conventional Medicine: Recent research has explored the potential for integrating VRT into conventional medical settings, such as hospitals and clinics, as a complementary therapy for various health conditions.

8. Long-Term Effects: Studies examining the long-term effects of VRT have shown promising results, indicating that regular VRT sessions may lead to sustained improvements in health and well-being over time.

9. Safety and Side Effects: Research has indicated that VRT is generally safe and well-tolerated, with minimal side effects reported. However, more research is needed to fully understand the safety profile of VRT.

10. Mechanisms of Action: Ongoing research is investigating the underlying mechanisms of action of VRT, including its effects on the nervous system, endocrine system, and immune system, to better understand how it produces its therapeutic effects.

Overall, research into Vertical Reflex Therapy (VRT) is continuing to grow, with promising developments indicating its potential benefits for a variety of health conditions.

Advanced Techniques and Applications of Vertical Reflex Therapy (VRT)

1. Neuro-Reflex Therapy:
- A specialized form of VRT that focuses on stimulating reflex points to address

neurological conditions, such as neuropathy, stroke recovery, and Parkinson's disease.

2. Meridian Reflexology Integration:

- Combining VRT with meridian therapy to stimulate specific meridians and acupoints through the feet and hands, based on traditional Chinese medicine principles.

3. Chakra Balancing:

- Using VRT to work with the body's chakras, or energy centers, to promote balance and harmony in the body's energy system.

4. Auricular Reflexology:

- Applying VRT techniques to the reflex points on the ears to stimulate corresponding areas of the body, similar to auricular acupuncture.

5. Lymphatic Drainage:

- Using VRT to stimulate reflex points associated with the lymphatic system to promote lymphatic drainage and detoxification.

6. Advanced Foot Mobilization Techniques:

- Incorporating gentle foot mobilization techniques into VRT to improve joint mobility and alignment.

7. Reflexology for Pregnancy and Postpartum:

- Developing specialized VRT protocols for pregnant women and new mothers to address specific concerns related to pregnancy and childbirth.

8. Sports Reflexology:

- Using VRT techniques to support athletes in their training and recovery by focusing on reflex points that can enhance performance and reduce the risk of injury.

9. Reflexology for Mental Health:

- Developing protocols for using VRT to support mental health, including stress reduction, anxiety management, and mood enhancement.

10. Integrative Reflexology:

- Integrating VRT with other complementary therapies, such as massage, acupuncture, and aromatherapy, to create comprehensive treatment plans for clients.

These advanced techniques and applications of Vertical Reflex Therapy (VRT) are expanding the scope of reflexology practice and offering new avenues for promoting health and well-being.

Continuing Education and Training in Vertical Reflex Therapy (VRT)

Continuing education and training are essential for reflexologists looking to enhance their skills and knowledge in Vertical Reflex Therapy (VRT).

Here are some ways to continue learning and growing in the field of VRT:

1. Advanced VRT Courses:

- Attend advanced VRT courses offered by reputable VRT organizations or instructors.

- These courses may cover topics such as advanced techniques, specialized protocols, and integrating VRT with other modalities.

2. Reflexology Conferences and Workshops:

- Attend reflexology conferences and workshops that feature VRT as a topic.

- These events often provide opportunities to learn from leading experts in the field and connect with other reflexologists.

3. Online Courses and Webinars:

- Take advantage of online courses and webinars that offer VRT training.
- These courses can be a convenient way to learn new techniques and concepts from the comfort of your own home.

4. Refresher Courses:

- Take refresher courses in VRT to review and reinforce your knowledge and skills.
- These courses can help you stay up-to-date with the latest developments in VRT practice.

5. Advanced Anatomy and Physiology Courses:

- Enhance your understanding of the human body by taking advanced anatomy and physiology courses.

- This knowledge can help you better understand the underlying mechanisms of VRT and how it affects the body.

6. Clinical Practice and Mentoring:

- Participate in clinical practice or mentoring programs where you can receive feedback and guidance from experienced VRT practitioners.
- This hands-on experience can help you refine your skills and gain confidence in your VRT practice.

7. Research and Literature Review:

- Stay informed about the latest research and literature on VRT by regularly reviewing journals, books, and articles in the field.

- This can help you stay current with the latest developments in VRT practice and theory.

8. Specialized Certifications:

- Consider pursuing specialized certifications in areas related to VRT, such as neuro-reflexology or meridian therapy.
- These certifications can help you expand your expertise and offer specialized services to your clients.

Continuing education and training are key to advancing your skills and knowledge in Vertical Reflex Therapy (VRT) and providing the best possible care to your clients.

CHAPTER 8

Vertical Reflex Therapy (VRT) for Specific Conditions

1. Chronic Pain Management: VRT can be effective in managing chronic pain conditions, such as lower back pain, neck pain, and arthritis. By stimulating reflex points associated with pain relief, VRT can help reduce pain levels and improve overall quality of life.

2. Stress and Anxiety: VRT is known for its relaxing and calming effects, making it beneficial for reducing stress and anxiety. By targeting reflex points associated with the nervous system and stress response, VRT can help promote relaxation and reduce feelings of anxiety.

3. Digestive Disorders: VRT can help improve digestive function by stimulating reflex points associated with the digestive system. This can help alleviate symptoms of digestive disorders such as bloating, constipation, and indigestion.

4. Sleep Disorders: VRT can be beneficial for improving sleep quality and addressing sleep disorders such as insomnia. By stimulating reflex points associated with relaxation and sleep, VRT can help promote restful sleep.

5. Immune System Support: VRT can help support the immune system by stimulating reflex points associated with the lymphatic system and immune response. This can help strengthen the immune system and improve overall health.

6. Hormonal Imbalance: VRT can help balance hormones by stimulating reflex points associated with the endocrine system. This can be beneficial for women experiencing hormonal imbalances related to menstruation, menopause, or thyroid issues.

7. Musculoskeletal Conditions: VRT can be effective in managing musculoskeletal conditions such as fibromyalgia, sciatica, and tendonitis. By stimulating reflex points associated with muscle and joint health, VRT can help reduce pain and improve mobility.

8. Neurological Conditions: VRT may be beneficial for neurological conditions such as neuropathy, stroke recovery, and Parkinson's disease. By stimulating reflex points associated with nerve function and brain health, VRT can help improve neurological symptoms and quality of life.

9. Pregnancy and Postpartum Support: VRT can be beneficial for pregnant women and new mothers by promoting relaxation, reducing stress, and addressing common pregnancy discomforts. By stimulating reflex points associated with reproductive health, VRT can help support a healthy pregnancy and postpartum recovery.

10. Overall Well-being and Preventive Care: VRT can be used as a preventive measure to maintain overall health and well-being. By stimulating reflex points throughout the body,

VRT can help promote balance, improve circulation, and support the body's natural healing abilities.

Using Vertical Reflex Therapy (VRT) for Pain Management

Vertical Reflex Therapy (VRT) can be a beneficial and effective modality for managing various types of pain. By stimulating reflex points on the feet or hands, VRT can help reduce pain levels, improve circulation, and promote relaxation.

Here's how VRT can be used for pain management:

1. Identifying Reflex Points: Reflexologists trained in VRT are skilled at identifying reflex points on the feet or hands that correspond to areas of the body experiencing pain.

2. Stimulating Reflex Points: Using specific techniques such as thumb walking, finger walking, or rotation, the reflexologist applies pressure to the reflex points associated with the painful area.

3. Pain Relief: The pressure applied to the reflex points helps stimulate the body's natural healing response, which can lead to pain relief and relaxation of the muscles.

4. Improving Circulation: VRT can help improve circulation to the painful area, which can reduce inflammation and promote healing.

5. Relaxation Response: The deep pressure applied during VRT can also trigger the body's relaxation response, which can help reduce stress and tension that may contribute to pain.

6. Holistic Approach: VRT takes a holistic approach to pain management, considering the interconnectedness of the body, mind, and spirit. This approach can help address underlying issues that may be contributing to pain.

7. Complementary Therapy: VRT can be used as a complementary therapy alongside other pain management techniques, such as medication, physical therapy, or acupuncture.

8. Individualized Treatment: Each VRT session is tailored to the individual, taking into account their specific pain symptoms and health history. This personalized approach can lead to more effective pain management outcomes.

Overall, VRT can be a valuable tool for managing pain and improving overall well-being. By stimulating reflex points on the feet or hands, VRT can help reduce pain levels, improve circulation, and promote relaxation, making it a holistic and effective approach to pain management.

Using Vertical Reflex Therapy (VRT) for Stress Relief and Relaxation

Vertical Reflex Therapy (VRT) is known for its ability to promote relaxation and reduce stress levels. By stimulating reflex points on the feet or hands, VRT can help activate the body's relaxation response, leading to a sense of calm and well-being.

Here's how VRT can be used for stress relief and relaxation:

1. Stimulating Reflex Points: Reflexologists trained in VRT use specific techniques to apply pressure to reflex points on the feet or hands that are associated with relaxation and stress relief.

2. Activating the Relaxation Response: The pressure applied during VRT helps activate the body's relaxation response, which can lead to a decrease in stress hormones and an increase in feel-good neurotransmitters like endorphins.

3. Promoting Circulation: VRT can help improve circulation to the feet and hands, which can promote relaxation and reduce tension in the body.

4. Reducing Muscle Tension: The deep pressure applied during VRT can help release tension in the muscles, leading to a feeling of relaxation and ease.

5. Improving Sleep Quality: VRT can help improve sleep quality by promoting relaxation and reducing stress levels, making it easier to fall asleep and stay asleep.

6. Complementary Therapy: VRT can be used as a complementary therapy alongside other stress-relief techniques, such as meditation, yoga, or massage.

7. Individualized Treatment: Each VRT session is tailored to the individual, taking into account their specific stress symptoms and health history. This personalized approach can lead to more effective stress relief outcomes.

8. Mind-Body Connection: VRT recognizes the connection between the mind and body, and aims to promote balance and harmony in both. By addressing both physical and emotional aspects of stress, VRT can help promote overall well-being.

Overall, VRT can be a valuable tool for promoting relaxation and reducing stress levels. By stimulating reflex points on the feet or hands, VRT can help activate the body's relaxation response, leading to a sense of calm and well-being.

Using Vertical Reflex Therapy (VRT) for Enhancing Overall Well-being

Vertical Reflex Therapy (VRT) is a holistic therapy that can be used to enhance overall well-being by promoting balance and harmony in the body. By stimulating reflex points on the feet or hands, VRT can help improve circulation, boost the immune system, and support the body's natural healing abilities.

Here's how VRT can be used to enhance overall well-being:

1. **Improving Circulation:** VRT can help improve circulation to the feet and hands, which can promote overall health and vitality.

2. Boosting the Immune System: By stimulating reflex points associated with the lymphatic system and immune response, VRT can help boost the immune system and improve resistance to illness.

3. Reducing Stress and Tension: VRT can help reduce stress levels and promote relaxation, which can have a positive impact on overall well-being.

4. Supporting the Body's Natural Healing Abilities: VRT stimulates the body's reflex points, which are believed to correspond to specific organs and systems in the body. By stimulating these points, VRT can help support the body's natural healing abilities.

5. Balancing Energy Flow: VRT aims to balance the body's energy flow, promoting a sense of harmony and well-being.

6. Holistic Approach: VRT takes a holistic approach to health and well-being, considering the interconnectedness of the body, mind, and spirit. This approach can help address underlying issues that may be impacting overall well-being.

7. Complementary Therapy: VRT can be used as a complementary therapy alongside other wellness practices, such as massage, acupuncture, or yoga, to enhance overall well-being.

8. Individualized Treatment: Each VRT session is tailored to the individual, taking into account their specific health goals and concerns. This personalized approach can lead to more effective outcomes.

Overall, VRT can be a valuable tool for enhancing overall well-being by promoting balance, harmony, and vitality in the body. By stimulating reflex points on the feet or hands, VRT can help improve circulation, boost the immune system, and support the body's natural healing abilities, leading to a greater sense of well-being.

CHAPTER 9

The Future of Vertical Reflex Therapy (VRT)

Vertical Reflex Therapy (VRT) has the potential to play an increasingly significant role in the field of complementary and alternative medicine. As the practice continues to evolve, several trends and developments are shaping the future of VRT:

1. Research and Evidence-Based Practice: There is a growing interest in conducting research studies to further validate the effectiveness of VRT. Continued research will help establish VRT as an evidence-based practice and enhance its integration into mainstream healthcare.

2. Integration into Healthcare Settings: VRT is increasingly being integrated into conventional healthcare settings, such as hospitals, clinics, and wellness centers. As awareness of VRT grows, more healthcare professionals may incorporate it into their practice as a complementary therapy.

3. Technological Advancements: Technology is playing an increasing role in VRT, with the development of tools and devices that can enhance the effectiveness of VRT techniques. These advancements may include biofeedback devices, virtual reality tools, and digital platforms for VRT training and education.

4. Specialized Training and Certification: As interest in VRT grows, there may be an increase in specialized training programs and certification courses for reflexologists interested in mastering VRT techniques. These programs will help ensure high standards of practice and quality care for clients.

5. Integration with Other Modalities: VRT is being integrated with other complementary modalities, such as massage therapy, acupuncture, and aromatherapy, to create comprehensive treatment plans for clients. This integrative approach can enhance the overall effectiveness of VRT and improve client outcomes.

6. Focus on Wellness and Prevention: VRT's holistic approach to health and wellness makes it well-suited for promoting wellness and preventing illness. As more people seek ways to maintain their health and prevent disease, VRT may become increasingly popular as a preventive healthcare practice.

7. Global Recognition and Adoption: VRT is gaining recognition and adoption around the world, with an increasing number of practitioners offering VRT services in various countries. This global recognition may lead to greater acceptance and integration of VRT into healthcare systems worldwide.

Overall, the future of VRT looks promising, with continued research, technological advancements, and integration into healthcare settings contributing to its growth and development. As VRT continues to evolve, it has the potential to become a widely accepted and valued practice in the field of complementary and alternative medicine.

Emerging Trends and Future Directions in Vertical Reflex Therapy (VRT)

1. Personalized Treatment Plans: The future of VRT may involve more personalized treatment plans based on individual needs and health goals. Reflexologists may use a combination of VRT techniques and other modalities to create customized treatment plans for each client.

2. Integration with Technology: Technology may play a larger role in VRT, with the development of tools and devices that can enhance the effectiveness of VRT techniques. This may include wearable devices, biofeedback tools, and digital platforms for VRT education and training.

3. Research and Evidence-Based Practice: There is a growing interest in conducting research studies to further validate the effectiveness of VRT. Future research may focus on specific conditions and populations to provide more evidence for the benefits of VRT.

4. Specialized Training and Certification: As interest in VRT grows, there may be an increase in specialized training programs and certification courses for reflexologists interested in mastering VRT techniques. These programs will help ensure high standards of practice and quality care for clients.

5. Integration into Healthcare Settings: VRT is increasingly being integrated into conventional healthcare settings, such as hospitals, clinics, and wellness centers. As awareness of VRT grows, more healthcare professionals may incorporate it into their practice as a complementary therapy.

6. Focus on Wellness and Prevention: VRT's holistic approach to health and wellness makes it well-suited for promoting wellness and preventing illness. As more people seek ways to maintain their health and prevent disease, VRT may become increasingly popular as a preventive healthcare practice.

7. Global Recognition and Adoption: VRT is gaining recognition and adoption around the world, with an increasing number of practitioners offering VRT services in various countries. This global recognition may lead to greater acceptance and integration of VRT into healthcare systems worldwide.

8. Continued Innovation: The future of VRT will likely involve continued innovation in techniques and approaches. Reflexologists may develop new VRT techniques or adapt existing techniques to better meet the needs of their clients.

Overall, the future of VRT looks promising, with emerging trends and developments that have the potential to further enhance its effectiveness and popularity as a complementary therapy for health and wellness.

Potential Advancements and Innovations in Vertical Reflex Therapy (VRT)

1. **Advanced Technology Integration:** As technology continues to advance, there may be opportunities to integrate VRT with cutting-edge technologies. For example, the development of virtual reality (VR) or augmented reality (AR) applications could enhance the VRT experience by providing visualizations or simulations of reflex points and their corresponding areas of the body.

2. **Biofeedback Devices:** The use of biofeedback devices could enhance the effectiveness of VRT by providing real-time feedback on the body's response to treatment. This could help reflexologists tailor their

techniques to each individual's needs and track progress over time.

3. Genetic and Biomarker Analysis: Advancements in genetic testing and biomarker analysis could lead to personalized VRT treatments based on an individual's genetic makeup and biomarker profile. This could help identify specific reflex points that may be particularly beneficial for each person.

4. Telehealth and Remote VRT: The use of telehealth technologies could allow for remote VRT sessions, expanding access to VRT for individuals who are unable to visit a reflexologist in person. This could be particularly beneficial for individuals in rural or underserved areas.

5. Robot-Assisted VRT: Robots equipped with VRT techniques could be developed to provide consistent and precise treatments. This could be especially useful in clinical settings where a high level of accuracy and repeatability is required.

6. Integration with Artificial Intelligence (AI): AI algorithms could be used to analyze data from VRT sessions and provide insights into the most effective treatment approaches for different conditions. This could help refine VRT techniques and improve outcomes for clients.

7. Nutrigenomics and VRT: The emerging field of nutrigenomics, which studies the interaction between nutrition and genetics, could be integrated with VRT to provide personalized dietary recommendations that complement VRT treatments.

8. Environmental and Lifestyle Factors:
Future advancements in VRT may involve a deeper understanding of how environmental and lifestyle factors impact health and how VRT can be used to address these factors. This could lead to more holistic and comprehensive treatment approaches.

Overall, the future of VRT holds exciting possibilities for advancements and innovations that could further enhance its effectiveness and accessibility as a complementary therapy for health and wellness.

Resources for Staying Updated on Vertical Reflex Therapy (VRT) Developments

1. VRT Organizations and Associations:

- The Vertical Reflex Therapy (VRT) website and social media channels provide updates on VRT developments, research, and events.

- The International Institute of Reflexology (IIR) offers courses and resources on VRT and reflexology in general.

2. Professional Journals and Publications:

- "Reflexions" is a journal published by the Association of Reflexologists (AoR) in the UK, which often includes articles on VRT and other reflexology topics.

- "Reflexology Research" is a peer-reviewed journal that publishes research on reflexology, including VRT studies.

3. Conferences and Workshops:

- The International Council of Reflexologists (ICR) organizes conferences and workshops where VRT developments are often discussed.
- The Reflexology Association of America (RAA) also hosts conferences and workshops that may cover VRT topics.

4. Online Forums and Communities:

- Joining online forums and communities dedicated to reflexology and VRT can be a great way to stay updated on developments and connect with other practitioners.

5. Continuing Education Courses:

- Taking continuing education courses in VRT can keep you informed about the latest techniques and approaches.

- Look for courses offered by reputable VRT organizations and instructors.

6. Research Databases:

- Accessing research databases such as PubMed can help you stay updated on the latest VRT research studies and findings.

7. Networking with Peers:

- Networking with other reflexologists and VRT practitioners can provide valuable insights and information on developments in the field.

By utilizing these resources, reflexologists can stay informed about the latest developments in VRT and continue to enhance their practice.

CHAPTER 10

Summary of Key Takeaways on Vertical Reflex Therapy (VRT)

1. VRT Basics: VRT is a reflexology technique that involves applying pressure to reflex points on the feet or hands while the limb is in a weight-bearing position, known as the "vertical" position. This approach is believed to enhance the body's response to treatment.

2. Benefits of VRT: VRT can promote relaxation, reduce stress, improve circulation, and support the body's natural healing abilities. It is used to address a wide range of conditions and promote overall well-being.

3. Techniques and Applications: VRT techniques include thumb walking, finger walking, and rotation, which are used to stimulate reflex points. VRT can be used as a standalone treatment or integrated with other complementary therapies.

4. Integration with Technology: The future of VRT may involve the integration of technology, such as biofeedback devices and virtual reality tools, to enhance the effectiveness of treatments and improve client outcomes.

5. Research and Evidence-Based Practice: There is a growing interest in conducting research studies to validate the effectiveness of VRT. Continued research will help establish VRT as an evidence-based practice and enhance its integration into mainstream healthcare.

6. Continuing Education and Training: Reflexologists interested in mastering VRT techniques can pursue specialized training and certification courses. These programs ensure high standards of practice and quality care for clients.

7. Global Recognition and Adoption: VRT is gaining recognition and adoption worldwide, with an increasing number of practitioners offering VRT services. This global recognition may lead to greater acceptance and integration of VRT into healthcare systems.

8. Future Directions: The future of VRT holds exciting possibilities, including personalized treatment plans, advanced technology integration, and research advancements. These developments have the potential to further enhance the effectiveness and accessibility of VRT as a complementary therapy.

Encouragement for Further Exploration and Practice of Vertical Reflex Therapy (VRT)

For those considering or already practicing Vertical Reflex Therapy (VRT), the journey holds great promise and potential for personal and professional growth.

Here are some encouraging words to inspire further exploration and practice:

1. Deepening Your Understanding: Embrace the opportunity to deepen your understanding of the human body's intricate reflex systems. Every session, every study, and every client interaction is a chance to expand your knowledge and expertise.

2. Impactful Healing: Remember the profound impact VRT can have on the lives of your clients. Your practice has the power to alleviate pain, reduce stress, and enhance overall well-being, making a meaningful difference in their lives.

3. Continuous Learning: Stay curious and open to new learning opportunities. The field of VRT is constantly evolving, and there's always more to discover and explore. Consider attending workshops, conferences, and courses to enhance your skills and knowledge.

4. Sharing Your Knowledge: Share your passion for VRT with others. Whether it's through teaching, writing, or simply sharing your experiences, your insights can inspire and educate others in the field.

5. Building Relationships: Cultivate strong relationships with your clients and colleagues. Your practice is not just about providing a service; it's about building trust, understanding, and connection with those you serve.

6. Embracing Challenges: Embrace challenges as opportunities for growth. Every setback or obstacle is a chance to learn and improve, ultimately making you a stronger and more resilient practitioner.

7. Personal Growth: Recognize the personal growth that comes from practicing VRT. As you help others heal and find balance, you may also experience your own transformation and self-discovery.

8. Contributing to the Field: Remember that your practice contributes to the broader field of reflexology and complementary medicine. Your dedication and commitment help elevate the profession and make VRT more widely recognized and respected.

In summary, the practice of Vertical Reflex Therapy is not just a profession, but a journey of discovery, healing, and personal growth. Embrace this journey with passion, dedication, and an open heart, and you will continue to make a positive impact on the lives of others and the field of reflexology as a whole.

Final Thoughts

As you embark on your journey with Vertical Reflex Therapy (VRT), remember that you are entering a field rich with potential for personal and professional growth. Your dedication to learning and practicing VRT has the power to transform lives, including your own.

As you explore the techniques and principles of VRT, take the time to acknowledge the pioneers and practitioners who have paved the way before you. Their dedication and passion have helped shape the field of reflexology and VRT into what it is today.

Always approach your practice with an open heart and mind, embracing each client and each session as a unique opportunity for healing and connection. Your commitment to your clients' well-being and your ongoing education will ensure that you continue to grow and evolve as a reflexologist.

Remember, too, to take care of yourself along the way. Self-care is essential for maintaining balance and perspective in your practice. As you nurture others, remember to nurture yourself as well.

In closing, I wish you success and fulfillment in your journey with VRT. May your practice be a source of healing, joy, and inspiration for yourself and those you serve.

Glossary of Vertical Reflex Therapy (VRT) Terms

1. Vertical Reflex Therapy (VRT): A reflexology technique where the hands or feet are worked in a weight-bearing position, believed to enhance the body's response to treatment.

2. Reflexology: A practice that involves applying pressure to specific points on the hands, feet, and ears to promote relaxation and healing in other parts of the body.

3. Reflex Points: Areas on the hands, feet, or ears that correspond to specific organs, glands, and other parts of the body.

4. Thumb Walking: A VRT technique where the thumb is used to apply pressure to reflex points, often in a walking motion.

5. Finger Walking: Similar to thumb walking, but using the fingers to apply pressure to reflex points.

6. Rotation: A VRT technique where the thumb or fingers are used to make circular movements on reflex points.

7. Lymphatic Reflex Points: Reflex points on the hands and feet that correspond to the lymphatic system, believed to help improve lymphatic drainage and immune function.

8. Endocrine Reflex Points: Reflex points on the hands and feet that correspond to the endocrine glands, believed to help balance hormone levels.

9. Nervous System Reflex Points: Reflex points on the hands and feet that correspond to the nervous system, believed to help reduce stress and promote relaxation.

10. Musculoskeletal Reflex Points: Reflex points on the hands and feet that correspond to the musculoskeletal system, believed to help relieve muscle tension and improve mobility.

11. Integration: The process of incorporating VRT into conventional healthcare settings or complementary therapy practices.

12. Biofeedback Devices: Devices that provide real-time feedback on the body's physiological responses, used to enhance VRT treatments.

13. Virtual Reality (VR) Tools: Tools that create a simulated environment, used in conjunction with VRT to enhance the treatment experience.

14. Nutrigenomics: The study of how nutrition impacts gene expression, potentially used in conjunction with VRT to provide personalized dietary recommendations.

15. Telehealth: The use of telecommunications technology to provide healthcare services remotely, potentially used to deliver VRT treatments to clients in remote locations.

16. Continuing Education: Ongoing training and education for reflexologists to stay updated on the latest VRT techniques and developments.

CONCLUSION

As we come to the end of this journey through the world of Vertical Reflex Therapy (VRT), I hope you've gained valuable insights into this transformative therapy and its potential to enhance your health and well-being. Throughout this handbook, we've explored the principles, techniques, and benefits of VRT, and I trust that you now have the knowledge and tools to integrate this powerful practice into your life.

A Holistic Approach to Health: VRT offers a holistic approach to health that addresses not only the physical body but also the mind and spirit. By stimulating reflex points in the weight-bearing feet and hands, VRT can help restore balance to the body's systems, promote relaxation, and enhance overall well-being.

Empowering Self-Care: One of the greatest strengths of VRT is its accessibility. Whether you're a trained reflexology practitioner or simply someone looking to improve your health, VRT can be easily integrated into your daily routine. By learning the techniques of VRT, you can empower yourself to take control of your health and well-being.

Continuing Your Journey: As you continue on your journey with VRT, I encourage you to explore the advanced techniques and applications of this therapy. Consider incorporating VRT into your professional practice or sharing it with others who may benefit from its healing effects. Stay curious, stay open-minded, and continue to explore the endless possibilities of VRT.

I invite you to take the knowledge and skills you've gained from this compendium and put them into practice. Begin your journey to balance and well-being today by incorporating VRT into your life. Whether you're seeking relief from pain, stress, or simply looking to enhance your overall health, VRT offers a natural and effective solution.

Thank You: Finally, I want to express my gratitude to you, the reader, for joining me on this journey. It has been a pleasure to share the world of VRT with you, and I hope that this compendium has inspired you to explore the incredible potential of Vertical Reflex Therapy.

Remember, the key to balance and well-being lies within you—unlock it with VRT.

Wishing you health, happiness, and balance on your journey ahead.